Dosage Calculations for Nursing Students: A Complete Guide

Mastering Medication Math for Nursing School and the NCLEX

Dr. David P. Zapencki, DNP, MSN/Ed, CNE, CCRN

Professional Development Publishing

ISBN (Paperback): 978-1-971135-00-7
ISBN (eBook): 978-1-971135-01-4

Published by Professional Development Publishing.

Preface

Medication administration is one of the most critical responsibilities a nurse will ever carry. Every dose calculated, every drip rate set, every syringe drawn represents a direct impact on patient safety. There is no room for error—and yet, dosage calculations remain one of the most challenging skills for nursing students to master.

This textbook was written with one goal in mind: to transform medication math from a source of anxiety into a source of confidence.

The chapters that follow take a deliberate, scaffolded approach. We begin with foundational concepts—the formulas, conversions, and safe-practice principles that form the bedrock of every calculation. From there, we progress through oral and parenteral medications, IV flow rates, critical-care drips, and pediatric dosing. Each chapter builds on the last, reinforcing core skills while introducing new complexity.

What sets this text apart is its emphasis on clinical reasoning. Nursing is not about memorizing formulas in isolation; it is about applying those formulas in real patient care scenarios. That is why you will find not only practice problems but also multi-step clinical scenarios, safe-dose range evaluations, and the kind of critical thinking questions you will encounter on the NCLEX and in your nursing career.

To the student reading this: medication math can be learned. It requires practice, patience, and a willingness to work through problems step by step. Do not skip ahead. Do not rush. Master each chapter before moving to the next. Use the practice problems. Check your work against the answer key. Understand not just *what* the answer is, but *why*.

Your future patients are counting on your accuracy. This book will help you develop the skills and confidence to deliver safe, precise medication administration every time.

Welcome to your journey toward mastery.

Dr. David P. Zapencki

Table of Contents

CHAPTER 1

Foundations of Medication Math

1.1 Overview: Why Medication Math Matters

Medication accuracy is essential to safe nursing practice. Every dose, every route, and every calculation affects patient outcomes. Nurses are responsible for preparing, administering, and evaluating medications, so fluency in medication math is foundational. Errors may occur when conversions are incorrect, when dosage forms are misunderstood, or when clinical context is not considered.

1.2 Core Methods of Dosage Calculation

Formula Method

Dose Desired (D) ÷ Dose on Hand (H) × Quantity (Q) = Amount to Give

Example: Order: 500 mg

Available: 250 mg tablets

500 ÷ 250 × 1 = 2 tablets

Ratio–Proportion Method

H : Q = D : X

Example: 250 mg : 1 tablet = 500 mg : X → X = 2 tablets

Dimensional Analysis (DA)

Example: 500 mg × (1 tablet / 250 mg) = 2 tablets

DA is especially helpful for IV flow rates, pediatric dosing, and critical-care titrations.

1.3 Units of Measurement

Common metric units include mg, g, mcg, mL, and L.

Key conversions:

- 1 g = 1,000 mg
- 1 mg = 1,000 mcg
- 1 L = 1,000 mL

Household conversions:

- 1 tsp = 5 mL
- 1 Tbsp = 15 mL
- 1 oz = 30 mL

1.4 Reading Medication Labels

Medication labels include:

- Drug name
- Dosage strength (e.g., 250 mg/5 mL)
- Dosage form
- Route (PO, IM, IV)
- Total volume
- Expiration date

1.5 Safe Practice Principles

- Always convert weight to kilograms
- Never round until the final step
- Use leading zeros (0.5 mg) but never trailing zeros (1.0 mg)
- Question doses outside expected ranges
- Always integrate clinical reasoning

1.6 Clinical Application Examples

Example 1

Order: 250 mg

Available: 125 mg/mL

250 ÷ 125 = 2 mL

Example 2

Order: 1 g

Available: 500 mg capsules

1 g = 1,000 mg

1,000 ÷ 500 = 2 capsules

Example 3

Order: 30 mg PO

Available: 15 mg tablets

30 ÷ 15 = 2 tablets

1.7 Practice Problems (20)

1. 500 mg; available 250 mg tablets
2. 1 g; available 500 mg capsules
3. Convert 2 g → mg
4. Convert 1,200 mg → g
5. 20 mg; available 10 mg/mL
6. 60 mg; available 30 mg tablets
7. 90 mg; available 15 mg/mL
8. Convert 0.5 L → mL
9. 12.5 mg; available 25 mg scored tablets
10. 200 mg; available 100 mg/mL
11. Convert 5 mg → mcg
12. Convert 4,500 mcg → mg
13. 80 mg; available 40 mg/5 mL
14. 15 mg; available 5 mg/mL
15. 300 mg; available 150 mg/mL
16. Convert 2.5 L → mL
17. Convert 3 tsp → mL
18. 250 mg; available 125 mg/mL
19. 0.25 g; available 250 mg tablets
20. 25 mg; available 12.5 mg tablets

CHAPTER 2

Medication Conversions

2.1 Overview

Medication conversions allow nurses to move between units, concentrations, and dosage forms with accuracy and confidence. Mastery of these foundational conversions is essential for safe practice—especially in pediatrics, critical care, and IV therapy.

This chapter reviews the most commonly used conversions in nursing practice, including metric, household, and apothecary units. It also explains when and why conversions matter clinically.

2.2 Metric Conversions

The metric system is the standard in healthcare. The most common units are:

- gram (g)
- milligram (mg)
- microgram (mcg)
- liter (L)
- milliliter (mL)

Key conversions:

- 1 g = 1,000 mg
- 1 mg = 1,000 mcg
- 1 L = 1,000 mL
- 1 mL = 1 cc (used interchangeably in clinical settings)

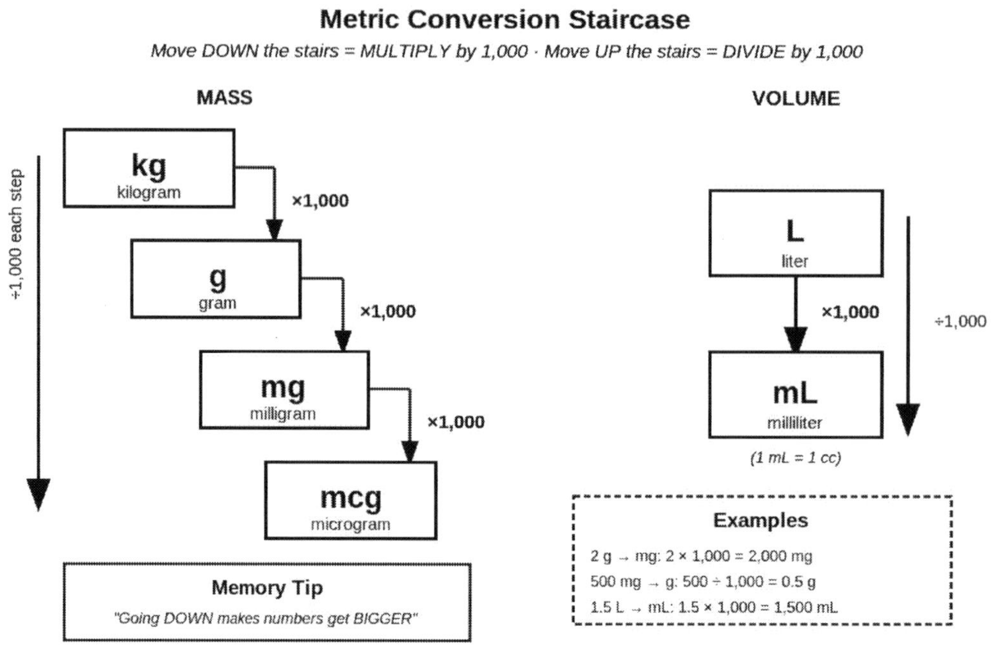

Figure 2.1 Metric conversion staircase for mass (kg, g, mg, mcg) and volume (L, mL) units.

Examples:

- Convert 3 g → mg
  3 g × 1,000 mg / 1 g = 3,000 mg
- Convert 2,500 mg → g
  2,500 mg ÷ 1,000 = 2.5 g

2.3 Household Conversions

Although the metric system is preferred, nurses will still encounter household measurements in medication orders and patient-reported dosing.

Key household conversions:

- 1 tsp = 5 mL
- 1 Tbsp = 15 mL
- 1 oz = 30 mL
- 1 cup = 240 mL

Examples:

- Convert 2 tsp → mL
  2 tsp × 5 mL = 10 mL
- Convert 1 oz → mL
  1 oz × 30 mL = 30 mL

2.4 Converting Between Systems

Many medication orders require converting between household and metric units.

Examples:

- 2 Tbsp → mL
  2×15 mL = 30 mL
- ½ cup → mL
  0.5×240 mL = 120 mL

2.5 Apothecary System (Less Commonly Used)

Some older medication references still use the apothecary system.

Common apothecary units:

- grain (gr)
- dram (dr)
- minim (min)

Approximate conversions you should know:

- 1 gr ≈ 60 mg
- 15 gr ≈ 1 g
- 1 dr ≈ 4 mL

Example:

- Convert 2 gr → mg
  2×60 mg = 120 mg

2.6 Converting Concentrations

Some medication orders require understanding concentration changes.

Example 1

Order: Give 0.5 g

Available: 250 mg tablets

Convert 0.5 g → mg

0.5 g × 1,000 mg = 500 mg

500 mg ÷ 250 mg = 2 tablets

Example 2

Order: Give 0.25 g

Available: 125 mg/mL solution

0.25 g = 250 mg

250 mg ÷ 125 mg/mL = 2 mL

2.7 Clinical Application Examples

Example 1

Order: Give 3 tsp of medication

Convert:

3 tsp × 5 mL = 15 mL

Example 2

Order: Give 2 oz of solution

Convert:

2 oz × 30 mL = 60 mL

Example 3

Order: Give 0.75 g PO

Available: 250 mg capsules

0.75 g = 750 mg

750 mg ÷ 250 mg = 3 capsules

2.8 Practice Problems (20)

1. Convert 4 g → mg
2. Convert 850 mg → g
3. Convert 3,000 mcg → mg

4. Convert 2.5 L → mL
5. Convert 8 tsp → mL
6. Convert 3 Tbsp → mL
7. Convert ½ cup → mL
8. Convert 2 oz → mL
9. Order: 0.5 g; available 250 mg tablets
10. Order: 1.2 g; available 400 mg capsules
11. Convert 3 gr → mg
12. Convert 15 gr → g
13. Convert 2 dr → mL
14. Convert 20 mL → Tbsp
15. Convert 45 mL → oz
16. Order: 0.25 g; available 125 mg/mL solution
17. Order: 0.75 g; available 250 mg capsules
18. Convert 90 mg → gr
19. Convert 1 oz → tsp
20. Convert 480 mL → cups

CHAPTER 3

Oral Medication Calculations

3.1 Overview

Oral medications are among the most commonly administered drugs in nursing practice. Tablets, capsules, liquids, and suspensions each require accurate dose calculations to ensure patient safety. This chapter builds on earlier concepts and focuses on the application of formula, ratio–proportion, and dimensional analysis methods for oral routes.

3.2 Solid Oral Dosage Forms

Many oral medications come in tablets or capsules. Nurses often calculate how many tablets to administer based on the ordered dose.

Formula:

Dose Desired (D) ÷ Dose on Hand (H) × Quantity (Q) = Tablets to Give

Example 1

Order: 650 mg PO

Available: 325 mg tablets

650 ÷ 325 × 1 = 2 tablets

Example 2

Order: 45 mg PO

Available: 15 mg tablets

45 ÷ 15 = 3 tablets

Scored tablets may be given in halves; unscored tablets should not be split unless pharmacy-approved.

3.3 Liquid Oral Medications

Liquid medications are measured in milliliters. Always verify concentration and total volume.

Example 1

Order: 80 mg PO

Available: 40 mg/5 mL

$80 \div 40 \times 5 = 10$ mL

Example 2

Order: 150 mg PO

Available: 75 mg/5 mL

$150 \div 75 \times 5 = 10$ mL

3.4 Measuring Oral Liquids

Key principles:

- Always use an oral syringe or calibrated measuring device
- Measure at eye level
- Do not use household utensils
- Shake suspensions thoroughly

Household-to-metric conversions (review):

- 1 tsp = 5 mL
- 1 Tbsp = 15 mL
- 1 oz = 30 mL

3.5 Multi-Step Oral Dose Calculations

Some medications require additional conversions before applying the formula method.

Example 1

Order: 1.2 g PO

Available: 400 mg tablets

Convert: 1.2 g = 1,200 mg

1,200 ÷ 400 = 3 tablets

Example 2

Order: 0.25 g PO

Available: 125 mg/5 mL

Convert: 0.25 g = 250 mg

250 ÷ 125 × 5 = 10 mL

3.6 Oral Syrups, Elixirs, and Suspensions

Nurses must understand different oral formulations:

- **Syrup** – thick, sweetened solution
- **Elixir** – clear, sweetened hydroalcoholic solution
- **Suspension** – particles dispersed in liquid; always shake well

Example

Order: 225 mg PO

Available: 75 mg/5 mL suspension

225 ÷ 75 × 5 = 15 mL

3.7 Clinical Application Examples

Example 1

Order: 15 mg PO

Available: 5 mg/mL

15 ÷ 5 = 3 mL

Example 2

Order: 600 mg PO

Available: 200 mg/5 mL

$600 \div 200 \times 5 = 15$ mL

Example 3

Order: 300 mg PO

Available: 150 mg tablets

$300 \div 150 = 2$ tablets

3.8 Practice Problems (20)

1. 45 mg ordered; available 15 mg tablets
2. 800 mg PO; available 400 mg tablets
3. 1.5 g; available 500 mg tablets
4. Convert 2 tsp → mL
5. Convert 1 oz → mL
6. 90 mg; available 30 mg/5 mL
7. 150 mg; available 75 mg/5 mL
8. 0.6 g; available 300 mg capsules
9. 25 mg; available 5 mg/mL
10. Convert 0.75 g → mg
11. 225 mg; available 75 mg/5 mL
12. 100 mg; available 50 mg tablets
13. Convert 3 Tbsp → mL
14. Convert ½ oz → mL
15. 10 mg; available 2 mg/mL
16. 75 mg; available 25 mg tablets
17. Convert 1.5 g → mg
18. 250 mg; available 125 mg tablets
19. Order 1 g PO; available 250 mg tablets
20. 500 mg; available 100 mg/5 mL

CHAPTER 4

Parenteral Medication Calculations

4.1 Overview

Parenteral medications are administered by injection and require heightened accuracy. In addition to dose calculations, nurses must understand syringe types, needle selection, reconstitution, and safe administration techniques. Errors in parenteral medication dosing can result in rapid and severe patient harm, making competence in this area essential.

This chapter reviews core principles and calculation methods for intradermal (ID), subcutaneous (SQ), intramuscular (IM), and intravenous (IV) injections.

4.2 Syringe Types and Measurement

Syringes come in several calibrated types:

- **Tuberculin (TB) syringes** – measured in tenths and hundredths of a milliliter (0.01 mL).
- **Insulin syringes** – marked in units (U-100 most common).
- **Standard syringes** – typically 1 mL, 3 mL, 5 mL, and 10 mL; marked in tenths.

Key principles:

- Always measure at the **leading edge** of the rubber plunger.
- Use the smallest syringe that can accurately deliver the dose.
- Insulin syringes must only be used for insulin.

Example

Order: 0.32 mL SQ

You must use a TB syringe (0.01 mL calibration).

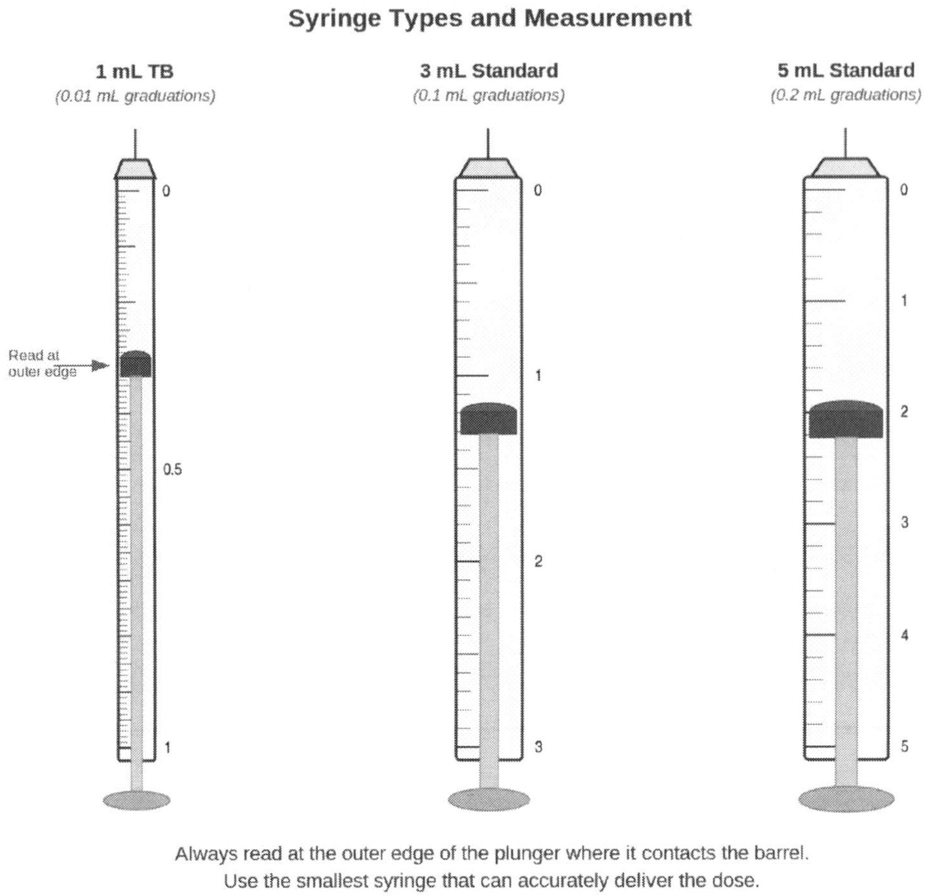

Figure 4.1 Comparison of 1 mL TB, 3 mL, and 5 mL syringes with their graduation markings.

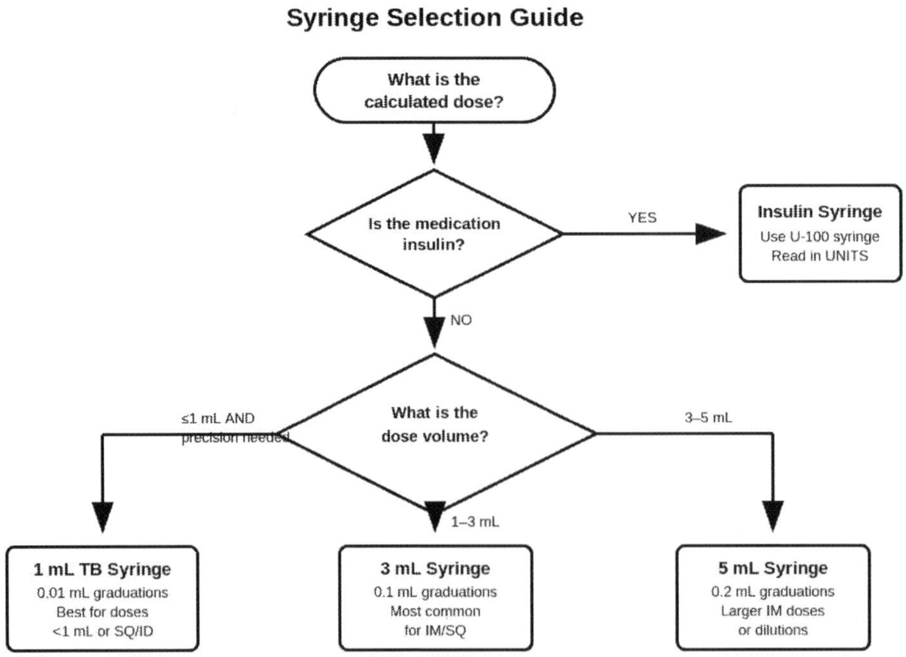

Figure 4.2 Syringe selection guide based on dose volume and medication type.

4.3 Needle Selection

Needles vary in gauge and length.

- **Gauge** = thickness; higher numbers mean thinner needles.
- **Length** = penetration depth needed for proper injection.

General guidelines (may vary by protocol):

- **ID:** 25–27 gauge, 3/8"–5/8"
- **SQ:** 25–30 gauge, 3/8"–5/8"
- **IM (deltoid):** 22–25 gauge, 1"
- **IM (vastus lateralis):** 22–25 gauge, 1–1.5"
- **IM (ventrogluteal):** 20–23 gauge, 1.5"

4.4 Injection Angles

Correct angle ensures proper medication deposition:

- **ID:** 5–15°
- **SQ:** 45–90° (depends on adipose tissue)
- **IM:** 90°

Example

If adipose tissue is minimal, SQ may require a 45° angle.

For obese patients, 90° may be appropriate.

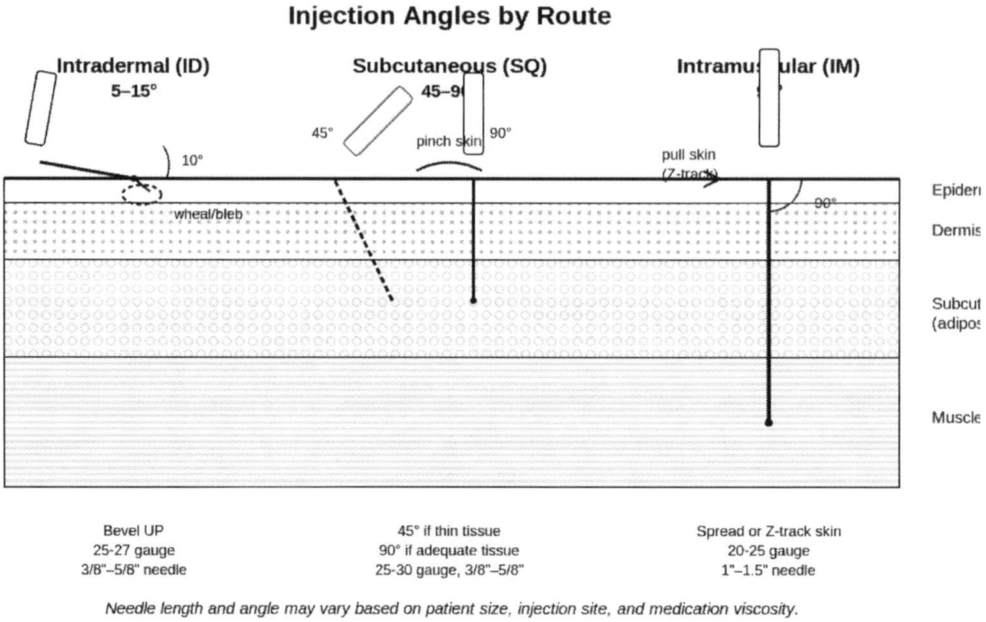

Figure 4.3 Injection angles for intradermal (ID), subcutaneous (SQ), and intramuscular (IM) routes.

4.5 Preparing Medications from Ampules

Key steps:

1. Tap the ampule top to move liquid down.
2. Wrap gauze around the neck and snap away from you.
3. Use a **filter needle** to withdraw solution.
4. Switch to a sterile administration needle before injection.

Example

Order: 4 mg IM

Available: 2 mg/mL ampule

4 ÷ 2 = **2 mL**

4.6 Preparing Medications from Vials

Vials may contain liquid medication or powder requiring reconstitution.

General steps:

1. Clean the rubber stopper with alcohol.
2. Inject an equal amount of air into the vial before withdrawing medication (for multi-dose vials).
3. Withdraw medication using sterile technique.

Example

Order: 10 mg IM

Available: 5 mg/mL

10 ÷ 5 = **2 mL**

4.7 Reconstitution of Medications

Some medications are supplied as powders and require dilution.

Example

Vial label:

- Powder contains 1 g drug
- Add 9.6 mL sterile water
- Final concentration: 100 mg/mL

Order: 250 mg IM

250 mg ÷ 100 mg/mL = **2.5 mL**

4.8 Z-Track Method for IM Injections

The Z-track method prevents irritation and leakage into subcutaneous tissue.

Steps:

1. Pull skin laterally 1–1.5 inches.
2. Insert needle at 90°.
3. Inject slowly.
4. Withdraw needle and release skin simultaneously.

Used especially for irritating IM medications (e.g., iron dextran).

4.9 Clinical Application Examples

Example 1

Order: 1.2 mL IM

Use a 3 mL syringe; round to the nearest tenth as needed.

Example 2

Order: 50 units insulin

Use a U-100 insulin syringe; administer **50 units** exactly (do not convert to mL).

Example 3

Order: 0.3 mL SQ

Available: 1 mg/1 mL

Dose: **0.3 mL** (no further conversion needed)

4.10 Practice Problems (20)

1. Order: 0.4 mL SQ; which syringe should you choose?
2. Order: 0.15 mL ID; available syringe markings?
3. Convert: 2 mL IM using 5 mg/mL solution → mg
4. Convert: 1.5 mL using 50 mg/mL solution → mg
5. Order: 75 mg IM; available 25 mg/mL → mL?
6. Choose appropriate gauge/length for a deltoid injection.
7. Choose appropriate gauge/length for ventrogluteal IM.
8. Order: 300 mg IM; available 100 mg/mL → mL?
9. Angle for SQ injection in a patient with minimal adipose tissue?
10. Angle for ID injection?
11. Order: 6 mg IM; available 2 mg/mL ampule → mL?
12. Order: 90 mg IM; available 30 mg/mL → mL?
13. Order: 1 g; available 500 mg/mL solution → mL?
14. Reconstituted vial: 200 mg/mL; order 50 mg → mL?
15. Identify correct syringe for 0.28 mL dose.
16. Identify correct needle gauge for SQ injection.
17. Identify correct gauge for thick IM medication.
18. Order: 20 units insulin; concentration U-100 → units given?
19. Order: 0.45 mL ID; which syringe?
20. Order: 900 mg; available 300 mg/mL → mL?

CHAPTER 5

IV Flow Rates & Infusions

5.1 Overview

Intravenous (IV) medications and fluids allow for rapid and precise delivery of treatment. Nurses must accurately calculate flow rates for both **manual gravity infusions** (gtt/min) and **electronic infusion pumps** (mL/hr). Miscalculations can result in underdosing, overdosing, fluid overload, or delayed treatment.

This chapter reviews IV flow rate formulas, drip factor selection, pump programming, manual vs. pump calculations, and clinical application problems.

5.2 Drip Factors (Manual Gravity Infusion)

Manual IV administration sets come with specific calibrated drip chambers. The drip factor appears on the tubing package.

Common drip factors:

- 10 gtt/mL (macrodrip)
- 15 gtt/mL (macrodrip)
- 20 gtt/mL (macrodrip)
- 60 gtt/mL (microdrip)

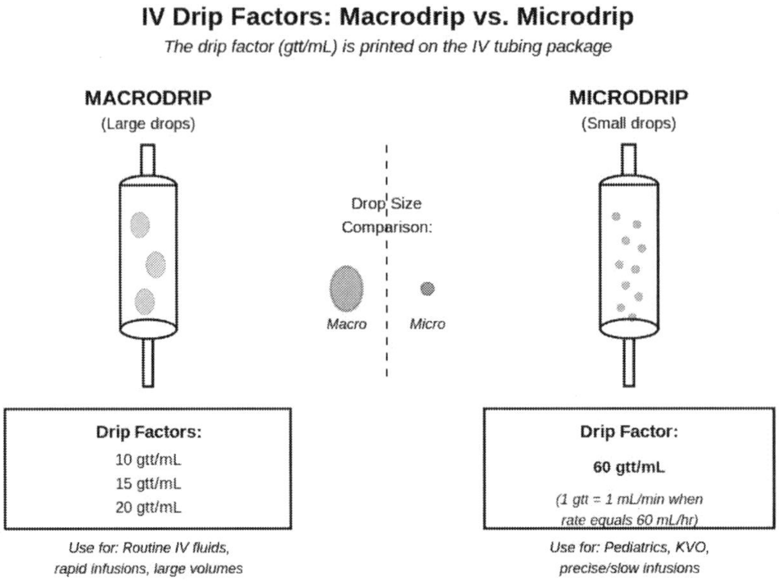

Figure 5.1 Macrodrip vs. microdrip IV tubing and their drip factors.

Key formula:

mL/hr → gtt/min

mL/hr × (gtt/mL) ÷ 60 = gtt/min

Example

Order: Infuse 1,000 mL over 8 hours using 15 gtt/mL tubing

Step 1: 1,000 ÷ 8 = 125 mL/hr

Step 2: 125 × 15 ÷ 60 = **31 gtt/min**

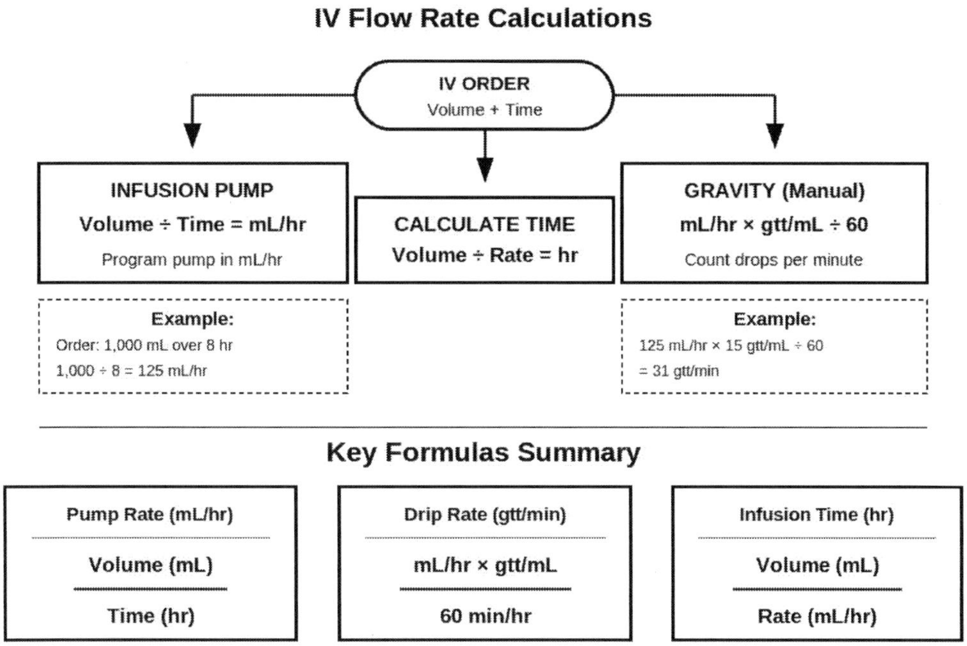

Figure 5.2 IV flow rate calculation formulas for infusion pumps and gravity drips.

5.3 Infusion Pumps (mL/hr)

Electronic infusion pumps are used whenever precise control is required.

Key formula:

mL to infuse ÷ hours = mL/hr

Example

Order: Infuse 500 mL over 4 hr

500 ÷ 4 = **125 mL/hr**

Another Example

Order: 75 mL/hr for 6 hr

Total infused = 75 × 6 = **450 mL**

5.4 Calculating Infusion Time

Sometimes the pump rate is known, but the nurse must calculate how long the infusion will run.

Formula:

Volume ÷ Rate = Time (hr)

Example

Order: Infuse 600 mL at 200 mL/hr

600 ÷ 200 = **3 hr**

5.5 IV Push (Bolus) Medications

IV push medications are given over short periods (e.g., 2–10 minutes). These require:

- precise dose calculation
- correct dilution volume
- correct administration rate

Example

Order: Give 4 mg IV over 2 minutes

Available: 2 mg/mL

4 ÷ 2 = **2 mL**, administered over **2 minutes**

5.6 IV Piggyback (IVPB) Medications

IVPB medications are secondary infusions connected to a primary line.

Example

Order: Administer 100 mg in 50 mL over 30 min

Rate = 50 mL ÷ 0.5 hr = **100 mL/hr**

Or, if via gravity using 20 gtt/mL tubing:

50 mL × 20 ÷ 30 = **33 gtt/min**

5.7 Titrated (Adjustable) Medications

These medications (e.g., dopamine, norepinephrine) are adjusted based on patient response.

Common formula (weight-based infusions):

(Dose × Weight × 60) ÷ Concentration = mL/hr

Example

Order: Dopamine 5 mcg/kg/min

Weight: 70 kg

Concentration: 400 mg in 250 mL

(5 × 70 × 60) = 21,000 mcg/hr = 21 mg/hr

Convert drug concentration:

400 mg ÷ 250 mL = 1.6 mg/mL

21 mg/hr ÷ 1.6 mg/mL = **13.1 mL/hr**

5.8 Heparin Infusions

Heparin drips may be ordered in units/hr or units/kg/hr.

Example

Order: 1,000 units/hr

Available: 25,000 units in 250 mL

Concentration = 25,000 ÷ 250 = 100 units/mL

1,000 ÷ 100 = **10 mL/hr**

5.9 Clinical Application Scenarios

Example 1

Order: 1,000 mL NS over 6 hr using 20 gtt/mL

1,000 ÷ 6 = 167 mL/hr

167 × 20 ÷ 60 ≈ **56 gtt/min**

Example 2

Order: 75 mL/hr for 8 hr

Total = **600 mL**

Example 3

Order: 50 mg in 25 mL over 15 minutes

Rate: 25 mL ÷ 0.25 hr = **100 mL/hr**

5.10 Practice Problems (20)

1. Infuse 500 mL over 5 hr (pump rate?).
2. Infuse 750 mL over 6 hr using 15 gtt/mL (gtt/min?).
3. 1,200 mL over 8 hr (pump rate?).
4. 90 mL/hr for 10 hr (total volume?).
5. Infuse 250 mL over 2 hr using 20 gtt/mL (gtt/min?).
6. Order: 100 mg in 50 mL over 1 hr (mL/hr?).
7. 1,000 mL over 4 hr (pump rate?).
8. 200 mL/hr for 3 hr (total volume?).
9. 1 L over 8 hr using 10 gtt/mL (gtt/min?).
10. Order 500 mL over 30 min using 15 gtt/mL (gtt/min?).
11. Dopamine: 5 mcg/kg/min; weight 80 kg; concentration 400 mg in 250 mL → mL/hr?
12. Heparin: 900 units/hr; concentration 100 units/mL → mL/hr?
13. Infuse 150 mL over 45 min (mL/hr?).
14. 60 mL/hr for 12 hr (total volume?).
15. 25 mL over 10 min using 60 gtt/mL (gtt/min?).
16. Order: 30 mg in 50 mL over 20 minutes (mL/hr?).
17. 2,000 mL over 24 hr (pump rate?).
18. Calculate infusion time: 800 mL at 200 mL/hr.
19. Order: 20 units/hr insulin; concentration 100 units/mL → mL/hr?
20. 40 mL over 30 minutes (mL/hr?).

CHAPTER 6

Critical-Care Medication Math

6.1 Overview

Critical-care medications are potent, fast-acting, and often weight-based. These medications include vasoactive drips, sedation infusions, inotropes, vasopressors, antiarrhythmics, and insulin infusions. Because their effects occur rapidly, precise calculation is essential. Even small errors can cause significant hemodynamic instability.

This chapter focuses on interpreting concentration labels, converting mg to mcg, calculating mcg/kg/min drips, preparing solutions, and adjusting infusion rates based on clinical response.

6.2 Review of Key Units

Critical-care infusions often use:

- **mcg/kg/min**
- **mcg/min**
- **mcg/hr**
- **units/hr** (e.g., insulin)
- **mL/hr** (pump settings)

Important conversions:

- 1 mg = 1,000 mcg
- 1 g = 1,000 mg
- 1 hour = 60 minutes

Example

Convert 5 mg → mcg

5 mg × 1,000 = **5,000 mcg**

6.3 Understanding Concentrations

Critical-care drips often come as "mg in mL."

Examples:

- Dopamine: 400 mg in 250 mL
- Norepinephrine: 4 mg in 250 mL
- Epinephrine: 1 mg in 250 mL
- Insulin: 100 units in 100 mL

To find concentration:

mg ÷ mL = mg/mL

Then convert mg/mL to mcg/mL if needed.

Example

Dopamine: 400 mg ÷ 250 mL = 1.6 mg/mL

1.6 mg/mL × 1,000 = **1,600 mcg/mL**

6.4 mcg/kg/min Formula

The universal formula used for all weight-based vasoactive infusions is:

(Dose × Weight × 60) ÷ Concentration = mL/hr

Where:

- Dose = mcg/kg/min ordered
- Weight = patient weight in kg
- 60 = minutes/hour
- Concentration = mcg/mL

Example

Order: Dopamine 5 mcg/kg/min

Weight: 70 kg

Concentration: 1,600 mcg/mL

Step 1: 5 × 70 × 60 = 21,000 mcg/hr

Step 2: 21,000 ÷ 1,600 = **13.1 mL/hr**

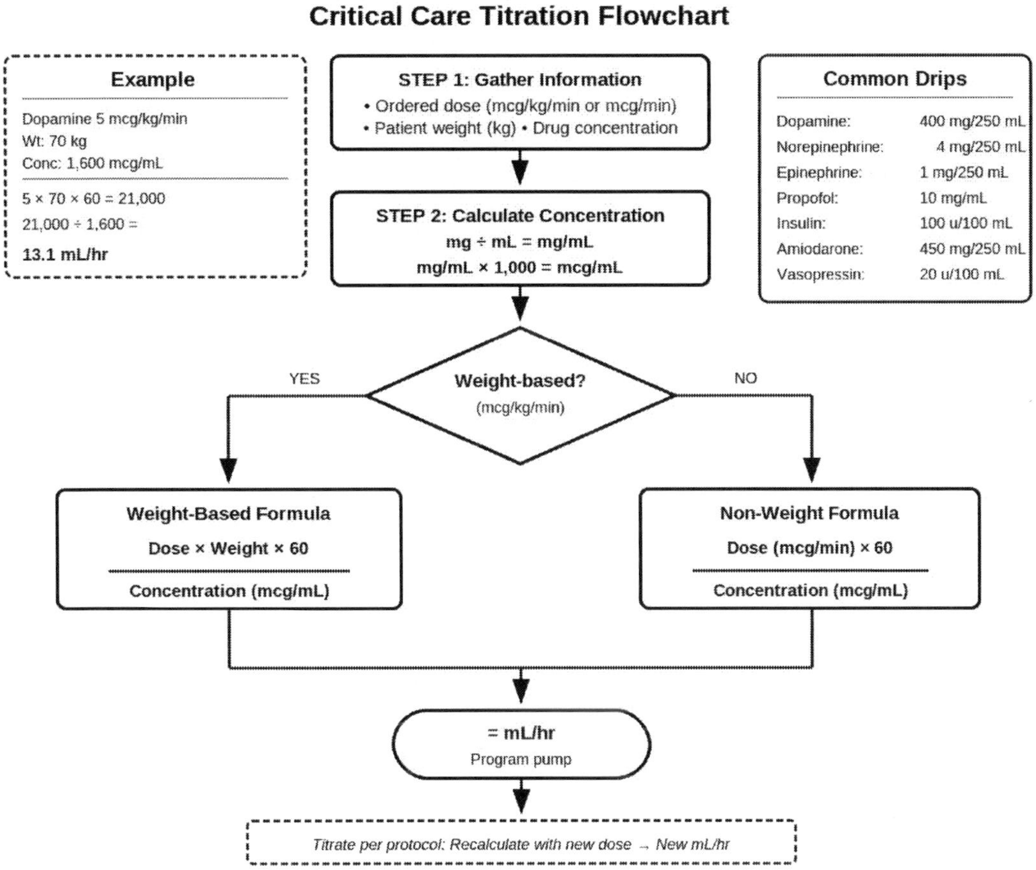

Figure 6.1 Critical care titration flowchart for calculating vasoactive drip rates.

6.5 Titration Adjustments

Many drips require frequent adjustments based on vitals, MAP, or protocol.

Example

Patient on norepinephrine at 6 mL/hr.

MAP goal: 65 mmHg; current MAP: 58 mmHg.

Increase per protocol: 1 mcg/min.

Calculate new mL/hr:

1. Convert ordered dose to mcg/hr:

   $1 \text{ mcg/min} \times 60 = 60 \text{ mcg/hr}$

2. If concentration is 16 mcg/mL:

   $60 \div 16 =$ **3.75 mL/hr increase**

New rate:

6 + 3.75 = **9.75 mL/hr**

6.6 Unit-Based Infusions (Insulin Example)

Example

Order: Insulin infusion at 5 units/hr

Available: 100 units in 100 mL

Concentration = 1 unit/mL

Rate = **5 mL/hr**

Another Example

Order: 12 units/hr

Rate = **12 mL/hr**

6.7 Antiarrhythmic Drips

Example: Amiodarone

Order: 1 mg/min for 6 hours

Concentration: 450 mg in 250 mL

Convert dose:

1 mg/min = 60 mg/hr

Concentration: 450 mg ÷ 250 mL = 1.8 mg/mL

60 ÷ 1.8 = **33.3 mL/hr**

6.8 Sedation Infusions (Propofol Example)

Example

Order: Propofol 20 mcg/kg/min

Weight: 80 kg

Concentration: 1,000 mcg/mL (10 mg/mL)

Step 1: 20 × 80 = 1,600 mcg/min

Step 2: 1,600 × 60 = 96,000 mcg/hr

Step 3: 96,000 ÷ 1,000 = **96 mL/hr**

6.9 Vasopressor Infusions (Norepinephrine Example)

Example

Order: 8 mcg/min

Concentration: 16 mcg/mL

8 × 60 = 480 mcg/hr

480 ÷ 16 = **30 mL/hr**

Another Example

Order: 0.05 mcg/kg/min

Weight: 90 kg

Dose: 0.05 × 90 = 4.5 mcg/min

Convert: 4.5 × 60 = 270 mcg/hr

270 ÷ 16 = **16.9 mL/hr**

6.10 Clinical Application Examples

Example 1

Order: Epinephrine 2 mcg/min

Concentration: 8 mcg/mL

Rate: 2 × 60 ÷ 8 = **15 mL/hr**

Example 2

Order: Vasopressin 0.03 units/min

Concentration: 20 units in 100 mL

Convert: 0.03 units/min × 60 = 1.8 units/hr

Rate: 1.8 ÷ 0.2 = **9 mL/hr**

Example 3

Order: Insulin 4 units/hr

Available: 1 unit/mL

Rate: **4 mL/hr**

6.11 Practice Problems (20)

1. Dopamine: 6 mcg/kg/min; wt 72 kg; conc 1,600 mcg/mL → mL/hr?
2. Norepinephrine: 4 mcg/min; conc 16 mcg/mL → mL/hr?
3. Propofol: 15 mcg/kg/min; wt 75 kg → mL/hr?
4. Dopamine: 10 mcg/kg/min; wt 60 kg → mL/hr?
5. Insulin: 8 units/hr; conc 1 unit/mL → mL/hr?
6. Amiodarone: 1 mg/min; conc 1.8 mg/mL → mL/hr?
7. Convert 0.2 mg/min → mg/hr
8. Convert 0.5 mg/min → mcg/hr
9. Vasopressin: 0.02 units/min → units/hr
10. Dopamine: 3 mcg/kg/min; wt 50 kg → mL/hr?
11. Propofol: 25 mcg/kg/min; wt 90 kg → mL/hr?
12. Norepinephrine: 12 mcg/min; conc 16 mcg/mL → mL/hr?
13. Insulin: 2 units/hr → mL/hr?
14. Milrinone: 0.5 mg/kg/min; wt 70 kg; conc 20 mg/100 mL → mL/hr?
15. Convert 1.2 mg/min → mcg/hr
16. Dopamine: 5 mcg/kg/min; wt 100 kg → mL/hr?
17. Vasopressin: 0.04 units/min → units/hr
18. Epinephrine: 3 mcg/min; conc 8 mcg/mL → mL/hr?
19. Norepinephrine: 6 mcg/min; conc 32 mcg/mL → mL/hr?
20. Heparin: 1,500 units/hr; conc 100 units/mL → mL/hr?

CHAPTER 7

Pediatric Dosage Calculations

7.1 Overview

Pediatric medication calculations require special attention due to differences in body size, organ maturity, fluid balance, and metabolic rate. Most pediatric doses are weight-based (mg/kg) and include safe-dose ranges to prevent harm. Because children are more sensitive to medication errors, accuracy is essential.

This chapter reviews weight conversions, mg/kg dosing, safe-dose range evaluation, pediatric fluid requirements, and clinical examples.

7.2 Weight Conversions

Pediatric weights must always be converted to kilograms (kg).

Key conversions:

- 1 kg = 2.2 lb
- lb → kg: weight in lb ÷ 2.2
- kg → lb: weight in kg × 2.2

Example

Child weighs 33 lb.

33 ÷ 2.2 = **15 kg**

Example

Infant weighs 9 kg.

9 × 2.2 = **19.8 lb**

7.3 mg/kg Dosing

Most pediatric medication orders are written in mg/kg.

Formula:

Ordered dose (mg/kg) × patient weight (kg) = mg to administer

Example

Order: 5 mg/kg

Weight: 12 kg

Dose: 5 × 12 = **60 mg**

Another Example

Order: 10 mg/kg

Weight: 4.5 kg

Dose: 10 × 4.5 = **45 mg**

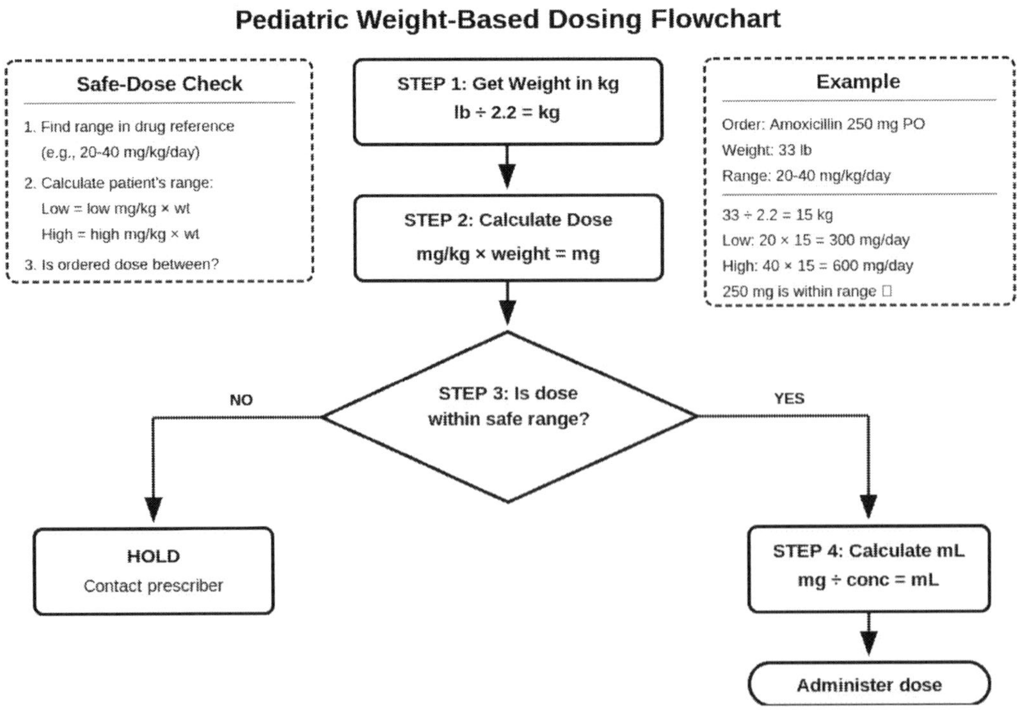

Figure 7.1 Pediatric weight-based dosing flowchart with safe-dose range verification.

7.4 Safe-Dose Ranges

Drug references include recommended pediatric ranges:

Example (amoxicillin)

- Safe-dose range: 20–40 mg/kg/day
- Patient weight: 18 kg

Calculate safe daily range:

- Low end: 20 × 18 = 360 mg/day
- High end: 40 × 18 = 720 mg/day

If an ordered dose exceeds the high end, it may be unsafe.

Example

Order: 500 mg/day

Range for 18 kg child: 360–720 mg/day → **Dose is safe**

7.5 Divided Doses

If a medication is ordered twice daily (BID), divide the total daily dose accordingly.

Example

Safe dose: 360–720 mg/day

Order: 500 mg/day BID

- Per-dose amount: 500 ÷ 2 = **250 mg per dose**

Check range: 360–720 mg/day is safe → BID order is acceptable.

7.6 Pediatric Liquid Medications

Many pediatric medications come as suspensions.

Example

Order: 60 mg

Available: 30 mg/5 mL

60 ÷ 30 × 5 = **10 mL**

Example

Order: 75 mg

Available: 15 mg/mL

75 ÷ 15 = **5 mL**

7.7 Pediatric Maintenance Fluids

A standard pediatric maintenance fluid formula is the **4–2–1 rule**:

- **First 10 kg:** 4 mL/kg/hr
- **Next 10 kg:** 2 mL/kg/hr
- **Each kg above 20 kg:** 1 mL/kg/hr

Example

Weight: 25 kg

- First 10 kg: 10 × 4 = 40
- Next 10 kg: 10 × 2 = 20
- Remaining 5 kg: 5 × 1 = 5

Total = **65 mL/hr**

Another Example

Weight: 8 kg

8 × 4 = **32 mL/hr**

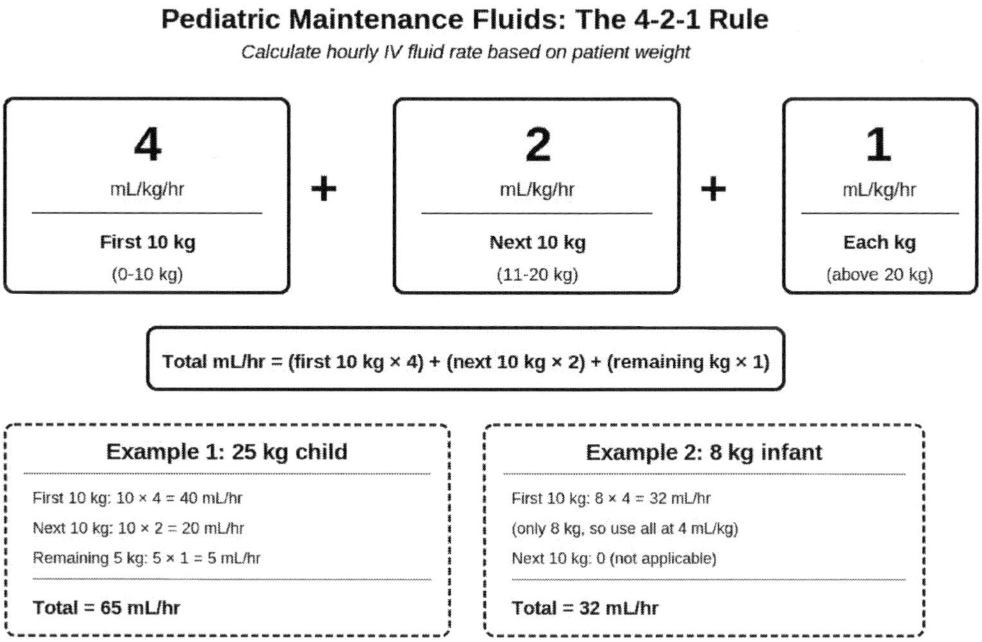

Figure 7.2 The 4-2-1 rule for calculating pediatric maintenance IV fluid rates.

7.8 Pediatric Fluid Bolus

Standard pediatric bolus:

- **20 mL/kg** of isotonic fluid

Example

Weight: 15 kg

Bolus: 15 × 20 = **300 mL**

7.9 Pediatric Clinical Application Examples

Example 1

Order: 6 mg/kg; weight 18 kg

6 × 18 = **108 mg**

Example 2

Order: 0.5 mL/kg; weight 12 kg

$0.5 \times 12 =$ **6 mL**

Example 3

Order: 4 mg/kg; weight 2.5 kg

$4 \times 2.5 =$ **10 mg**

Example 4

Order: 20 mL/kg bolus; weight 9 kg

$20 \times 9 =$ **180 mL**

7.10 Practice Problems (20)

1. Convert 44 lb → kg
2. Convert 9.2 kg → lb
3. Order: 6 mg/kg; weight 16 kg → mg?
4. Order: 4 mg/kg; weight 3.5 kg → mg?
5. Order: 10 mg/kg/day; weight 12 kg → daily mg?
6. Order: 12 mg/kg/day; weight 20 kg → daily mg?
7. Safe-dose range: 15–30 mg/kg/day; weight 10 kg → safe range?
8. Order: 500 mg/day; weight 10 kg → safe?
9. Liquid: 20 mg/mL; order 60 mg → mL?
10. Suspension: 30 mg/5 mL; order 90 mg → mL?
11. Maintenance fluids: 18 kg → mL/hr?
12. Maintenance fluids: 12 kg → mL/hr?
13. Bolus: 20 mL/kg; weight 22 kg → mL?
14. 7 mg/kg dose; weight 14 kg → mg?
15. 0.8 mL/kg; weight 16 kg → mL?
16. Safe-dose check: 25 mg/kg/day; weight 6 kg; order 200 mg/day
17. Convert 28 lb → kg
18. Order: 2 mg/kg; weight 2.2 kg → mg?
19. Bolus: 20 mL/kg; weight 3 kg → mL?
20. Maintenance fluids: 25 kg → mL/hr using 4–2–1 rule

CHAPTER 8

Advanced Clinical Scenarios

8.1 Overview

Advanced clinical dosage calculations require nurses to synthesize multiple skills: interpreting complex medication orders, integrating weight-based dosing, evaluating safe-dose ranges, calculating multiple routes (IV, PO, IM), adjusting infusion rates, and applying clinical reasoning to determine whether a dose is safe, appropriate, or requires clarification.

This chapter presents multi-step, realistic nursing scenarios similar to those encountered in clinical practice and Next Generation NCLEX-style questions.

8.2 Multi-Step Adult Scenarios

These problems require using combinations of conversions, safe-dose checks, and route-specific calculations.

Scenario 1

Order: Morphine 6 mg IV q2h PRN.

Available: Morphine 10 mg/mL vial.

Patient also receives morphine 2 mg/hr via PCA.

Question: How many mL do you administer for the PRN dose?

Calculation: 6 mg ÷ 10 mg/mL = **0.6 mL**

Scenario 2

Order: Cefazolin 1.5 g IVPB over 30 min.

Available: 1.5 g in 50 mL.

Rate: 50 mL ÷ 0.5 hr = **100 mL/hr**

Scenario 3

Order: Metoprolol 50 mg PO BID.

Available: 25 mg tablets.

Dose per administration: 50 ÷ 25 = **2 tablets**

8.3 Multi-Step Pediatric Scenarios

Pediatric problems require mg/kg dosing PLUS safe-dose range checks.

Scenario 1

Weight: 18 kg

Order: Acetaminophen 15 mg/kg/dose q6h

Dose: 15 × 18 = **270 mg per dose**

If available: 160 mg/5 mL → (270 ÷ 160) × 5 = **8.4 mL**

Scenario 2

Weight: 9 kg

Safe-dose range: 20–40 mg/kg/day

Order: 200 mg/day

Range: 180–360 mg/day → **Dose is safe**

Scenario 3

Weight: 32 lb

Convert weight: 32 ÷ 2.2 = **14.5 kg**

Order: 4 mg/kg

Dose: 4 × 14.5 = **58 mg**

8.4 Mixed Route Scenarios

These require calculating doses for more than one route in a single scenario.

Scenario 1

Order: Ondansetron 0.15 mg/kg IV prior to chemotherapy

Weight: 40 kg

Dose: 0.15 × 40 = **6 mg**

Available: 2 mg/mL → 6 ÷ 2 = **3 mL**

Scenario 2

Order: Atropine 0.02 mg/kg IM

Weight: 18 kg

Dose: 0.02 × 18 = **0.36 mg**

Available: 0.4 mg/mL → 0.36 ÷ 0.4 = **0.9 mL**

8.5 Advanced Dimensional Analysis (DA)

These problems combine several conversions in one calculation.

Example

Order: 2 mcg/kg/min

Weight: 75 kg

Available: 400 mg in 250 mL

Step 1: Convert concentration

400 mg = 400,000 mcg

400,000 mcg ÷ 250 mL = **1,600 mcg/mL**

Step 2: Calculate dose per hour

2 × 75 × 60 = 9,000 mcg/hr

Step 3: Calculate mL/hr

9,000 ÷ 1,600 = **5.6 mL/hr**

8.6 High-Alert Medication Scenarios

Certain medications (e.g., insulin, heparin, vasopressors) require special attention.

Scenario 1 — Insulin Infusion

Order: 3 units/hr

Available: 100 units in 100 mL

Concentration: 1 unit/mL

Rate: **3 mL/hr**

Scenario 2 — Heparin

Order: 1,200 units/hr

Available: 25,000 units in 250 mL

Concentration: 100 units/mL

Rate: 1,200 ÷ 100 = **12 mL/hr**

Scenario 3 — Norepinephrine

Order: 10 mcg/min

Concentration: 16 mcg/mL

Convert dose: 10 × 60 = 600 mcg/hr

Rate: 600 ÷ 16 = **37.5 mL/hr**

8.7 Fluid Balance & Intake/Output Scenarios

Some dosage decisions depend on fluid status.

Scenario 1

Patient intake is 2,100 mL for the last 24 hours; output is 1,800 mL.

Net balance = **+300 mL**

Scenario 2

Order: Add additional 40 mL/hr to correct deficit over 8 hours.

Additional volume = 40 × 8 = **320 mL**

8.8 Clinical Practice Set (20 Advanced Problems)

1. Ceftriaxone 75 mg/kg/day; weight 22 kg → daily dose?
2. Dopamine 8 mcg/kg/min; wt 70 kg; conc 1,600 mcg/mL → mL/hr?
3. Convert 1.5 g → mg; order 1.5 g over 45 minutes → mL/hr if in 100 mL?
4. Weight 55 lb → kg; order 10 mg/kg → mg?
5. Insulin 7 units/hr; concentration 1 unit/mL → mL/hr?
6. Amiodarone 360 mg in 200 mL over 6 hr → mL/hr?
7. Order: 0.2 mg/kg; weight 9 kg → mg?
8. Order: 20 mL/kg bolus; weight 28 kg → mL?
9. 1 g in 250 mL over 2 hr → pump rate?
10. Norepinephrine 6 mcg/min; conc 16 mcg/mL → mL/hr?
11. Pediatric safe range: 10–30 mg/kg/day; weight 14 kg → safe range?
12. Order: 600 mg/day; range safe?
13. Dopamine 3 mcg/kg/min; wt 50 kg → mL/hr?
14. Convert 33 lb → kg; order 5 mg/kg → mg?
15. 40 mg; available 10 mg/5 mL → mL?
16. Heparin 1,500 units/hr; conc 100 units/mL → mL/hr?
17. Propofol 10 mcg/kg/min; wt 85 kg → mL/hr?
18. 250 mL IV to infuse over 75 minutes → mL/hr?
19. 2 g medication; available 500 mg tablets → tablets?
20. Pediatric maintenance fluids: 22 kg → using 4-2-1 rule → mL/hr?

CHAPTER 9

Comprehensive Practice Sets

9.1 Overview

This chapter provides comprehensive practice across all major dosage calculation domains, including oral medications, parenteral routes, IV pump and drip-rate calculations, pediatric mg/kg dosing, safe-dose range evaluation, and critical-care medication math. These problems mimic the range and complexity of questions seen on exams, in clinical rotations, and on the NCLEX.

Each section contains a variety of question formats and difficulty levels.

9.2 Oral Medication Calculations

1. Order: 450 mg PO; available 150 mg tablets → tablets?
2. 1.2 g PO; available 400 mg tablets → tablets?
3. Order: 75 mg; available 25 mg/5 mL → mL?
4. Order: 500 mg; available 125 mg/5 mL → mL?
5. 0.6 g PO; available 300 mg capsules → capsules?
6. Convert 3 tsp → mL
7. Convert 2 Tbsp → mL
8. 30 mg PO; available 10 mg tablets → tablets?
9. 325 mg; available 65 mg/mL → mL?
10. Convert 1 oz → mL

9.3 Parenteral Medication Calculations

11. Order: 0.4 mL SQ; which syringe is appropriate?

12. Order: 0.15 mL ID; syringe choice?
13. 60 mg IM; available 30 mg/mL → mL?
14. 2 mL IM of 25 mg/mL → mg?
15. Correct angle for SQ injection in thin adult?
16. Correct gauge/length for deltoid IM injection?
17. 75 mg IM; available 25 mg/mL → mL?
18. Order: 3 mg IM; available 1 mg/mL → mL?
19. Reconstitution: vial 1 g powder; add 9 mL → conc?
20. Order: 250 mg from 100 mg/mL solution → mL?

9.4 IV Flow Rates & Pump Calculations

21. Infuse 1,000 mL over 8 hr (pump rate?).
22. 250 mL over 2 hr using 20 gtt/mL → gtt/min?
23. 75 mL/hr for 6 hr → total volume infused?
24. Infuse 500 mL over 4 hr → mL/hr?
25. 1,200 mL over 10 hr → mL/hr?
26. Infuse 100 mL over 30 min → mL/hr?
27. 50 mL over 20 min using 60 gtt/mL → gtt/min?
28. Infuse 800 mL at 200 mL/hr → time?
29. IVPB: 50 mL over 30 min → mL/hr?
30. 1,000 mL over 6 hr using 15 gtt/mL → gtt/min?

9.5 Pediatric Dosage Calculations

31. Weight: 44 lb → kg?
32. Weight: 9.5 kg → lb?
33. Order: 6 mg/kg; weight 16 kg → mg?
34. Order: 10 mg/kg; weight 4.5 kg → mg?
35. Safe-dose range: 20–40 mg/kg/day; weight 18 kg → safe range?
36. Order: 300 mg/day; safe?
37. Maintenance fluids: 14 kg → mL/hr?

38. Maintenance fluids: 25 kg → mL/hr?
39. Bolus: 20 mL/kg; weight 12 kg → mL?
40. Order: 0.2 mL/kg; weight 22 kg → mL?

9.6 Advanced & Critical-Care Calculations

41. Dopamine: 5 mcg/kg/min; wt 75 kg; conc 1,600 mcg/mL → mL/hr?
42. Norepinephrine: 6 mcg/min; conc 16 mcg/mL → mL/hr?
43. Insulin: 7 units/hr; conc 1 unit/mL → mL/hr?
44. Amiodarone: 1 mg/min for 6 hr; conc 1.8 mg/mL → mL/hr?
45. Propofol: 20 mcg/kg/min; wt 80 kg; conc 1,000 mcg/mL → mL/hr?
46. Vasopressin: 0.04 units/min; convert to units/hr
47. Heparin: 1,500 units/hr; conc 100 units/mL → mL/hr?
48. Calculate 0.5 mg/min → mcg/hr
49. Dopamine: 3 mcg/kg/min; wt 50 kg → mL/hr?
50. Norepinephrine: 12 mcg/min; conc 32 mcg/mL → mL/hr?

9.7 Integrated Clinical Scenarios

51. Patient weighs 32 lb. Convert to kg; order 5 mg/kg PO → mg?
52. Order: 1 g IV over 45 min; available 100 mL → mL/hr?
53. Order: 12 mg/kg/day divided BID; weight 18 kg → mg/dose?
54. Drip: 1 mg/min; conc 1.8 mg/mL → mL/hr?
55. Reconstituted vial: 200 mg/mL; order 50 mg → mL?
56. Weight: 10 kg; safe-dose range 10–30 mg/kg/day → safe range?
57. Order: 800 mL NS at 125 mL/hr → time?
58. 250 mL over 20 min using 20 gtt/mL → gtt/min?
59. 0.5 mg/kg; weight 9 kg → mg?
60. 1,000 units/hr heparin; conc 100 units/mL → mL/hr?

9.8 Summary

This comprehensive practice set brings together every dosage calculation skill covered in this text. Mastery of these problems ensures strong preparation for exams, clinical practice, and NCLEX-style medication safety questions.

CHAPTER 10

Answer Key & Rationales

10.1 Overview

This chapter provides detailed answers and rationales for all practice problems in Chapters 1 through 9. Rationales reinforce safe-practice reasoning, demonstrate correct calculation pathways, and highlight common errors to avoid.

10.2 Chapter 1 Answers — Foundations of Medication Math

1. 500 mg ÷ 250 mg = **2 tablets**
2. 1 g = 1,000 mg; 1,000 ÷ 500 = **2 capsules**
3. 2 g × 1,000 = **2,000 mg**
4. 1,200 mg ÷ 1,000 = **1.2 g**
5. 20 mg ÷ 10 mg = **2 mL**
6. 60 mg ÷ 30 mg = **2 tablets**
7. 90 mg ÷ 15 mg = **6 mL**
8. 0.5 L × 1,000 = **500 mL**
9. 12.5 mg ÷ 25 mg = **0.5 tablet**
10. 200 mg ÷ 100 mg = **2 mL**
11. 5 mg × 1,000 = **5,000 mcg**
12. 4,500 mcg ÷ 1,000 = **4.5 mg**
13. 80 mg ÷ 40 mg × 5 = **10 mL**
14. 15 mg ÷ 5 mg = **3 mL**
15. 300 mg ÷ 150 mg = **2 mL**
16. 2.5 L × 1,000 = **2,500 mL**

17. 3 tsp × 5 mL = **15 mL**

18. 250 mg ÷ 125 mg = **2 mL**

19. 0.25 g = 250 mg → 250 mg ÷ 250 mg = **1 tablet**

20. 25 mg ÷ 12.5 mg = **2 tablets**

10.3 Chapter 2 Answers — Medication Conversions

1. 4 g × 1,000 = **4,000 mg**

2. 850 mg ÷ 1,000 = **0.85 g**

3. 3,000 mcg ÷ 1,000 = **3 mg**

4. 2.5 L × 1,000 = **2,500 mL**

5. 8 tsp × 5 mL = **40 mL**

6. 3 Tbsp × 15 mL = **45 mL**

7. 0.5 × 240 = **120 mL**

8. 2 oz × 30 = **60 mL**

9. 500 mg ÷ 250 mg = **2 tablets**

10. 1.2 g = 1,200 mg; 1,200 ÷ 400 = **3 capsules**

11. 3 gr × 60 mg = **180 mg**

12. 15 gr ≈ **1 g**

13. 2 dr × 4 mL = **8 mL**

14. 20 mL ÷ 15 mL = **1.33 Tbsp**

15. 45 mL ÷ 30 mL = **1.5 oz**

16. 0.25 g = 250 mg; 250 ÷ 125 = **2 mL**

17. 0.75 g = 750 mg; 750 ÷ 250 = **3 capsules**

18. 90 mg ÷ 60 mg ≈ **1.5 gr**

19. 1 oz = **6 tsp**

20. 480 mL ÷ 240 mL = **2 cups**

10.4 Chapter 3 Answers — Oral Medication Calculations

1. 45 mg ÷ 15 mg = **3 tablets**

2. 800 mg ÷ 400 mg = **2 tablets**

3. Convert: 1.5 g = 1,500 mg; 1,500 ÷ 500 = **3 tablets**

4. 2 tsp × 5 = **10 mL**

5. 1 oz × 30 = **30 mL**

6. 90 ÷ 30 × 5 = **15 mL**

7. 150 ÷ 75 × 5 = **10 mL**

8. 0.6 g = 600 mg; 600 ÷ 300 = **2 capsules**

9. 25 ÷ 5 = **5 mL**

10. 0.75 g = **750 mg**

11. 225 ÷ 75 × 5 = **15 mL**

12. 100 ÷ 50 = **2 tablets**

13. 3 Tbsp × 15 = **45 mL**

14. 0.5 oz × 30 = **15 mL**

15. 10 ÷ 2 = **5 mL**

16. 75 ÷ 25 = **3 tablets**

17. 1.5 g = **1,500 mg**

18. 250 ÷ 125 = **2 tablets**

19. 1 g = 1,000 mg; 1,000 ÷ 250 = **4 tablets**

20. 500 ÷ 100 × 5 = **25 mL**

10.5 Chapter 4 Answers — Parenteral Calculations

1. **TB syringe**

2. **TB syringe** (0.01 mL calibration)

3. 2 mL × 5 mg/mL = **10 mg**

4. 1.5 mL × 50 mg/mL = **75 mg**

5. 75 ÷ 25 = **3 mL**

6. **22–25 gauge, 1"**

7. **20–23 gauge, 1.5"**

8. 300 ÷ 100 = **3 mL**

9. **45°**

10. **5–15°**

11. 6 ÷ 2 = **3 mL**

12. 90 ÷ 30 = **3 mL**
13. 1 g = 1,000 mg; 1,000 ÷ 500 = **2 mL**
14. 50 mg ÷ 200 mg/mL = **0.25 mL**
15. **TB syringe**
16. **25–30 gauge**
17. **20–23 gauge** (thicker meds need lower gauge numbers)
18. **20 units** (insulin syringe; 1:1 units)
19. **TB syringe**
20. 900 ÷ 300 = **3 mL**

10.6 Chapter 5 Answers — IV Flow Rates & Infusions

1. 500 ÷ 5 = **100 mL/hr**
2. 750 ÷ 6 = 125 mL/hr; 125 × 15 ÷ 60 = **31 gtt/min**
3. 1,200 ÷ 8 = **150 mL/hr**
4. 90 × 10 = **900 mL**
5. 250 ÷ 2 × 20 ÷ 60 = **42 gtt/min**
6. 100 ÷ 1 = **100 mL/hr**
7. 1,000 ÷ 4 = **250 mL/hr**
8. 200 × 3 = **600 mL**
9. 1,000 ÷ 8 × 10 ÷ 60 = **21 gtt/min**
10. 500 ÷ 0.5 × 15 ÷ 60 = **250 gtt/min**
11. (5 × 80 × 60) = 24,000; 24,000 ÷ 1,600 = **15 mL/hr**
12. 900 ÷ 100 = **9 mL/hr**
13. 150 ÷ 0.75 = **200 mL/hr**
14. 60 × 12 = **720 mL**
15. 25 × 60 ÷ 60 = **25 gtt/min**
16. 30 ÷ 0.333 = **90 mL/hr**
17. 2,000 ÷ 24 = **83 mL/hr**
18. 800 ÷ 200 = **4 hr**
19. 20 units; concentration 1 unit/mL → **20 mL/hr**
20. 40 ÷ 0.5 = **80 mL/hr**

10.7 Chapter 6 Answers — Critical-Care Medication Math

1. $(6 \times 72 \times 60) \div 1{,}600 =$ **16.2 mL/hr**
2. $4 \times 60 \div 16 =$ **15 mL/hr**
3. $15 \times 75 \times 60 \div 1{,}000 =$ **67.5 mL/hr**
4. $(10 \times 60 \times 60) \div 1{,}600 =$ **22.5 mL/hr**
5. **8 mL/hr**
6. $60 \div 1.8 =$ **33.3 mL/hr**
7. $0.2 \times 60 =$ **12 mg/hr**
8. 0.5 mg/min $= 0.5 \times 60 =$ 30 mg/hr → **30,000 mcg/hr**
9. $0.02 \times 60 =$ **1.2 units/hr**
10. $(3 \times 50 \times 60) \div 1{,}600 =$ **5.6 mL/hr**
11. $(25 \times 90 \times 60) \div 1{,}000 =$ **135 mL/hr**
12. $12 \times 60 \div 16 =$ **45 mL/hr**
13. **2 mL/hr**
14. $(0.5 \times 70 \times 60) =$ 2,100 mg/hr → $2{,}100 \div 20 =$ **105 mL/hr**
15. $1.2 \times 60 \times 1{,}000 =$ **72,000 mcg/hr**
16. $(5 \times 100 \times 60) \div 1{,}600 =$ **18.8 mL/hr**
17. $0.04 \times 60 =$ **2.4 units/hr**
18. $3 \times 60 \div 8 =$ **22.5 mL/hr**
19. $6 \times 60 \div 32 =$ **11.25 mL/hr**
20. $1{,}500 \div 100 =$ **15 mL/hr**

10.8 Chapter 7 Answers — Pediatric Dosage Calculations

1. $44 \div 2.2 =$ **20 kg**
2. $9.5 \times 2.2 =$ **20.9 lb**
3. $6 \times 16 =$ **96 mg**
4. $4 \times 3.5 =$ **14 mg**
5. $10 \times 12 =$ **120 mg/day**
6. $12 \times 20 =$ **240 mg/day**

7. 15–30 × 10 = **150–300 mg/day**

8. 500 mg/day → **unsafe** (exceeds 300 mg/day)

9. 60 ÷ 20 = **3 mL**

10. 90 ÷ 30 × 5 = **15 mL**

11. 4–2–1 rule: 14 kg → 4 × 10 + 2 × 4 = **48 mL/hr**

12. 4–2–1: 12 kg → 4 × 10 + 2 × 2 = **44 mL/hr**

13. 20 × 12 = **240 mL**

14. 7 × 14 = **98 mg**

15. 0.8 × 16 = **12.8 mL**

16. 25 × 6 = 150 mg/day → order 200 mg/day → **unsafe**

17. 28 ÷ 2.2 = **12.7 kg**

18. 2 × 2.2 = **4.4 mg**

19. 20 × 3 = **60 mL**

20. 4–2–1: 25 kg → 4 × 10 + 2 × 10 + 1 × 5 = **65 mL/hr**

10.9 Chapter 8 Answers — Advanced Clinical Scenarios

1. 75 mg/kg/day; 22 kg → **1,650 mg/day**

2. (8 × 70 × 60) ÷ 1,600 = **21 mL/hr**

3. 1.5 g = 1,500 mg → 100 mL over 45 min = **133 mL/hr**

4. 55 lb ÷ 2.2 = 25 kg → 10 × 25 = **250 mg**

5. **7 mL/hr**

6. 200 mL ÷ 6 = **33.3 mL/hr**

7. 0.2 × 9 = **1.8 mg**

8. 20 × 28 = **560 mL**

9. 250 mL ÷ 2 hr = **125 mL/hr**

10. 6 × 60 ÷ 16 = **22.5 mL/hr**

11. 10–30 × 14 = **140–420 mg/day**

12. Order 600 mg/day → **unsafe**

13. (3 × 50 × 60) ÷ 1,600 = **5.6 mL/hr**

14. 33 ÷ 2.2 = 15 kg → 5 × 15 = **75 mg**

15. 40 ÷ 10 × 5 = **20 mL**

16. 1,500 ÷ 100 = **15 mL/hr**

17. (10 × 85 × 60) ÷ 1,000 = **51 mL/hr**

18. 250 mL ÷ 1.25 hr = **200 mL/hr**

19. 2,000 mg ÷ 500 mg = **4 tablets**

20. 4–2–1: 22 kg → 4 × 10 + 2 × 10 + 1 × 2 = **62 mL/hr**

10.10 Summary

These rationales reinforce safe calculation methods, provide error-prevention tips, and guide clinical decision-making related to medication math across a wide range of patient populations and clinical contexts.

Quick Formula Reference

This reference summarizes the most commonly used formulas in nursing dosage calculations.

Metric Conversions (Chapter 2)

1 kg = 2.2 lb | 1 g = 1,000 mg | 1 mg = 1,000 mcg | 1 L = 1,000 mL

Dosage Calculation (Chapters 3-4)

Desired ÷ Have × Vehicle = Amount to give

IV Flow Rates (Chapter 5)

Pump rate: Volume (mL) ÷ Time (hr) = mL/hr

Drip rate:mL/hr × gtt/mL ÷ 60 = gtt/min

Infusion time: Volume (mL) ÷ Rate (mL/hr) = hours

Drip factors: Macrodrip = 10, 15, or 20 gtt/mL | Microdrip = 60 gtt/mL

Critical Care Drips (Chapter 6)

Weight-based:(Dose × Weight × 60) ÷ Concentration (mcg/mL) = mL/hr

Non-weight:(Dose × 60) ÷ Concentration (mcg/mL) = mL/hr

Pediatric Calculations (Chapter 7)

Weight conversion:lb ÷ 2.2 = kg

Weight-based dose:mg/kg × weight (kg) = mg

Safe-dose range: Low mg/kg × wt = low end | High mg/kg × wt = high end

4-2-1 Rule (maintenance IV fluids):

First 10 kg: 4 mL/kg/hr
Next 10 kg: 2 mL/kg/hr
Each kg above 20: 1 mL/kg/hr

Made in United States
Orlando, FL
06 November 2026

90281938R20037